YOUR KNOWLEDGE HAS VALUE

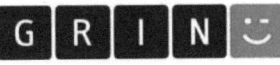

Green synthesis of silver Nanoparticles and its method development and validation by UV spectroscopy in bulk pharmaceuticals

U. M. Patel

Bibliographic information published by the German National Library:

The German National Library lists this publication in the National Bibliography; detailed bibliographic data are available on the Internet at http://dnb.dnb.de.

ISBN: 9783346983718
This book is also available as an ebook.

© GRIN Publishing GmbH
Trappentreustraße 1
80339 München

Print and binding: Books on Demand GmbH, Norderstedt, Germany
Printed on acid-free paper from responsible sources.

The present work has been carefully prepared. Nevertheless, authors and publishers do not incur liability for the correctness of information, notes, links and advice as well as any printing errors.

GRIN web shop: https://www.grin.com/document/1419236

GREEN SYNTHESIS OF SILVER NANOPARTICLES AND ITS METHOD DEVELOPMENT AND VALIDATION BY UV SPECTROSCOPY IN BULK PHARMACEUTICALS

U.M. PATEL[1]

[1]Department of Quality Assurance (PG), Sanjivani College of Pharmaceutical Education and Research, Kopargaon, Maharashtra, India.

1

Silver Nanoparticle has been recognized as safe inorganic, antibacterial, nontoxic agent. Conventional synthesis of Silver Nanoparticle can generate toxic waste during the reaction process hence, this paper the green synthesis approach used and for synthesis of silver nanoparticle by using *Datura metel* leaf extract as a reducing agent. The change in colour of silver nitrate solution from colourless to brown was visual identification for formation of Silver Nanoparticle and shown the absorption at 447 nm. The synthesized Silver Nanoparticle were of size 180 nm analyse by SEM and further characetrised by FTIR where carboxylic peak was obtained at 1675 cm^{-1} as well as presence of alcoholic group and polyphenols. Further validated method was developed and linearity was found to be 0.995 and % RSD of validation parameters were found to be within the limit <2%. A simple, lab scale, rapid, accurate, precised and sensitive spectroscopic method has been developed and validated as per ICH guideline for synthesized silver nanoparticle in bulk pharmaceuticals by UV vis spectrophotoscopy and which is applicable for routine analysis.

Keyword : Silver nanoparticle, *Datura metel* leaves, UV spectrophotometer, method development, validation, ICH guideline.

Silver nanoparticles, one of the most important noble metals. Silver nanoparticles (Ag-NPs) are known to have fungicidal effects and antimicrobial activity[1]. Silver and its related compounds has low toxicity for the animal cells whereas as the high toxicity for the microorganisms like bacteria and fungi. These synthesis of metal nanoparticle that too via green synthesis offers many advantages hence it is beign the recent area of research[3]. There is an increasing commercial demand for nanoparticles due to their wide applicability in various areas such as electronics , biology, chemistry and medicine. Recently, Ag NPs as well as various silver-based compounds containing the ionic silver (Ag+) or metallic silver (Ag^0) exhibiting antimicrobial activity have been synthesized. Antibacterial activity of the silver-containing materials is widely applicable, for example, in medicine to reduce infections in burn treatment and arthroplasty, as well as to prevent bacteria colonization on prostheses, catheters, vascular grafts, dental materials, stainless steel materials, and human skin. Although chemical and physical methods may successfully produce pure, well-defined nanoparticles, these methods are quite expensive and potentially dangerous to the environment. The convential method include use of the reducing agent along with the passivator which will prevent agglomeration of metallic nanoparticle and synthesized the nanoparticle in the stable form. But for large scale synthesis of metallic nanoparticle mercapto, thiourea are majorily used as passivator which are further responsible for producing toxic waste and harm the environment severly. Further the conventional approach of synthesis of metallic nanoparticles majorily leads to absorb some of the toxic chemicals on surface that leads to huge adverse effects upon its application. Hence, the environmental friendly procedures are required to synthesized the nanoparticle with desired size and shape without generating any toxic waste[2].Use of biological

3

organisms such as microorganisms, bacteria , fungi, and plant extract or plant biomass could be an alternative to chemical and physical methods for the production of nanoparticles in an ecofriendly manner that is going through green synthesis. The advantages of using plants for the synthesis of nanoparticles are that the plants are easily available and safe to handle and possess a large variety of active agents that can promote the reduction of silver ions[3,13]. Synthesis of Ag NPs by economic, eco-friendly simple route of green/biosynthesis of plant extract methods.

In this study, we report the synthesis of Ag NPs by green synthesis process using *Datura metel* leaf extract as reducing agent[2]. The final products characteristics were studied – optical, structural, surface morphology and elemental analysis. Green chemistry should aim at minimizing waste, minimizing energy use, employing renewable materials, and applying methods that minimize risk. The three main concepts for the preparation of nanoparticles in a green synthesis approach are the choice of the solvent medium (preferably water), an environmentally friendly reducing agent, and a nontoxic material for the stabilization of the nanoparticles[3]. The plant extract to be used for synthesis of nanoparticle contains biomolecules , which has dual action of reduction and as capping agent that leads to the formation of the stable silver nanoparticle. This biomolecules are phenolics, terpenoids, aminoacidsflavones etc[14].

The goal of the research was to synthesised Ag NPs by using plant extract i.e green synthesis approach which is coast effective, simple, non-toxic approach. Along with its method validation by UV spectrophotometeric method. UV-Visible validation method has been developed for their analysis. Quantification of the medicinal substance using UV spectrophotometer is done by preparing solution in the transparent solvent and measuring it's absorbance at the suitable wavelength by scanning under appropriate range. The wavelength normally selected is wavelength of where the sample has shown maximum absorption (λmax) Ideally, concentration should be adjusted to give the absorbance of approximately 0.9, that mean it should obey Beers Lamberts law [22].

As the formulations are available without combinations of any drugs, there is a need for coming up with analytical method which is simple, sensitive, rapid and accurate for estimation of Ag NPs in pure form and in pharmaceutical preparations . Therefore, the aim of the present work is to synthesized Ag NPs via green synthesis and development of lab scale UV Sphectrophotometric analytical method for routine analysis of formulation containing Ag NPs with or without combination and in bulk pharamaceuticals.. This validated UV method being used is rapid, accurate and precise for validation of Ag NPs in bulk pharmaceuticals[5].

MATERIALS AND METHODS:

Materials:

Ag NPs were synthesized in house by green synthesis using *Datura metel* leaves. *Datura metel* leaves were freshly collected from medicinal arden and authenticated by Dr N.G. Sutar Department of Pharmacognosy. Methanol and Silver Nitrate used were of the analytical grade and purchase from Mordern industries and selected as solvent system and synthesis purpose.

Method for synthesis of Ag NPs:

Datura metel leaves were freshly collected. To remove the soil and other contaminants present on the surface of fresh leaves, thoroughly washed with de-ionized water. After the wash, 10 g of leaves were cut into the small pieces and then soaked into 100 mL de-ionized water. These leaves were continuously stirred at 60 °C for 10 min and further filtered to get the extract. The plant extract was stored in refrigerator at 4 °C for the further use. 5 mL leaf extract was added drop by drop with 9 mM aqueous solution of silver nitrate (Ag NO$_3$). The reaction mixture of Ag NO$_3$ and leaf extract was stirred for 15 min to get colloidal solution of brown colour. The reduction process of Ag$^+$ ions to Ag^0 takes place, completely within the period of 15 min and observed visually by varying the initial colour of the reaction mixture from colourless to dark brown[2].

Characterization of synthesized Ag NPs:

The optical absorption spectrum was obtained using UV–vi spectrophotometer Shimadzu model 1650 .the scanning must be done from 300 -800nm for the aliquot of solution of the silver nanoparticle. Fourier transform infrared (FTIR) spectrum was measured using FTIR, Infinity. Shimadzu-8400. Before sampling of synthesized Ag NPs it is necessary for background scanning of FTIR. It was done between 400cm^{-1} to 4000cm^{-1}. The interaction between proteins and AgNPs along the functional group present can be analyzed by FTIR. Morphology of the sample was observed by scanning electron microscope of STIC at Kochi University Kerala, India

Method development:

Spectroscopic analysis was carried out using Double beam Shimadzu recording UV-Visible Spectrophotometer of model 1650 with 10 mm path length matched quartz cells was used for analytical purpose.

Preparation of Standard Stock Solution:

Stock solution of Ag NPs was prepared by dissolving 100mg of Ag NPs in 20 ml of methanol and sonicated for 45 minutes and further 80 ml water was added to it to adjust the volume up to 100 ml. And its aliquots were transferred in a series of 10 ml volumetric flasks in varying fractions and their volumes were made with methanol to prepare different standard dilutions.

Preparation of Working solution:

The aliquots were transferred in a series of 10 ml volumetric flasks in varying fractions and their volumes were made with methanol to prepare different standard dilutions. The sample was further scanned by a UV-VIS Spectrophotometer in the range of 300 – 800 nm, using methanol as a blank. The wavelength corresponding to the maximum absorbance (λmax) was found to be 447 nm.

Method Validation:

Validation of the method was carried out as per the International Conference on Harmonization (ICH) guidelines

Q2 (R1) (ICH, 2005) . And accordingly the parameters evaluated were:

Specificity
Linearity
Accuracy
Precision
Limit of detection
Limit of quantification
Ruggedness

Specificity:

Solutions of standard and sample were prepared as per working solution test procedure and further scanning for UV spectra was carried out. UV peak of standard and sample should be identical.

Linearity and range:

Six points calibration curve were obtained in a concentration range from 100-660 μg/ml for Ag NPs. The response was found to be linear in the investigation concentration range and the linear regression equation with correlation coefficient was obtained.

Accuracy:

To check the accuracy of the proposed method, recovery studies were carried out 50, 100 and 150% of the test concentration as per ICH guidelines. The recovery study was performed in triplicate at each level. The result of the recovery studies are reported in Table 4 .

Precision:

Precision of the analytical method is ascertained by carrying out the analysis as per the procedure and as per normal weight taken for analysis. Repeat the analysis six times. Average. Standard deviation, Relative standard deviation and % RSD calculated.

Interday and Intraday precision:

The Interday and intraday precision was determined by spiking standard solution on the same day and on different days at different time intervals respectively (six replicates). The results of the same are presented in Table 6 and 7.

Limit of detection:

Solutions of specific concentrations were prepared five times (five sets)[8] within range of calibration. The detection limit of an individual analytical procedure is the lowest amount of analyte in a sample, which can be detected, but not necessarily quantitated as an exact value[7].

$$L.O.D. = 3.3(SD/S) \ (9)$$

Where; SD is the standard deviation of y-intercept of the calibration curve, and S is the mean slope of five calibration curves[8].

Limit of quantification:

Solutions of specific concentrations were prepared five times (five sets)[8] within range of calibration. The quantitation limit is generally determined by the analysis of samples with known concentrations of analyte and by establishing the minimum level at which the analyte can be quantified with acceptable accuracy and precision.

$$LOQ = 10 \times SD/S$$

Where; SD is the standard deviation of y-intercept of the calibration curve, and S is the mean slope of five calibration curves[8].

Ruggedness:

It expresses the precision within laboratories variations like different analyst. Ruggedness of the method was assessed by spiking the standard 6 times with different analyst by using same equipment. The results of the same are presented in Table 7 and 8.

RESULTS

Synthesis of Ag NPs:

The theoretical yield was calculated considering the molecular weight of silver nitrate and Ag NPs. The theoretical yield was 0.996g and practical yield was found to be 0.756g . The percentage yield of synthesized Ag NPs was found to be 76%.

Spectrum Analysis:

Colloidal brown suspension of reaction mixture of silver nitrate solution and leaf extract shown the formation of Ag NPs. These brown colour solution is primary visual identification for the formation of the silver nanoparticle. The brown colour of solution was due to surface plasma resonance. Due to formation of silver crystals in reaction mixture,surface plasma resonance peak emerged at 447nm of wavelength analysed by UV vis spectroscopy. (Fig 1) and (fig 2) proves the formation of nanoparticle

FTIR Analysis:

FTIR Analysis was studied verify whether the required functional group are are their in synthesized Ag NPs. FTIR peak of AgNPs is reported in Table 1 and FTIR spectrum in (fig 3). The absorption peak located at 1046 cm^{-1} is for −C-O stretching vibrations of alcoholic groups. The peak emerged at 1387 cm^{-1} is due to −C-O-C stretching . The stretching vibrations at 1110 and 1460 cm^{-1} are attributed to hydroxyl functional groups in polyphenols and phenols, respectively. The presence of stretching vibration at 1675 cm^{-1} representing that Ag NPs is bounded to proteins via carboxylate group. The stretching vibration of −C-C- in aromatic ring causes an absorption peak at 1561 cm^{-1}. All these stretching vibrations and bends exhibit that proteins, carboxylic acids, alcoholic groups and polyphenols are bounded along with Ag NPs. This indicate that the phenolic content of plant extract has prevent the aggregation of the silver nanoparticle.

Surface Morphological studies:

The SEM image confirms that the Ag NPs are in nanoscale, particle are of size rang 180 nm as shown in (fig 4).

Method Validation:
The results are found to be within limits and results are summarized in Table 2.

Validation Parameter:

Specificity:

The UV peak of standard Ag NPs was found to be at 450 nm. The peak of synthesized silver nanopaticle was found to be 447 nm in methanol. Hence, peak obtained are identical.

Linearity and range:

Linearity of an analytical method is its ability, within a given range, to obtain test results that are directly, or through a mathematical transformation, proportional to concentration of analyte. Range of Ag NPs was found to be 160-660µg/ml and calibration curve was plotted, regression coefficient was found to be 0.995. The standard graph is reported in Table 3.

Accuracy:

The % recovery was found to be 97.7 $\pm$ 0.48%. The % RSD was found to be within the limit < 2%. The results are reported in Table 4.

Precision:

The precision was studied for intraday as well as interday and % RSD was found to be within limit < 2%, for intraday 0.98% and for interday 0.32%. the results are reported in Table 5 and 6.

Limit of detection(LOD):

The minimum quantity of Ag NPs detected is reported as LOD. From the data obtained LOD was found to be 18.15 µg/ml.

Limit of quantification(LOQ):

The minimum quantity of Ag NPs to be quantified is reported as LOQ. From the data obtained LOQ was found to be 55 µg/ml.

Ruggedness:

The % RSD was fond to be 1.23% which is within the limit. The results were reported in Table 7 and 8.

DISCUSSION

Using green synthesis, Ag NPs were synthesized from *Datura metel* leaf extract. Plant extract contain biomolecules which acts as reducing agent and capping agent which convert Ag^{3+} into Ag^0 and forms stable AgNPs. Synthesis was found to be efficient in terms of reaction time and stability of synthesized nanoparticle with 76 % of yield obtained via green synthesis apporach. Synthesized Ag NPs where further characterized by UV spectroscopy and showed absorbance at 447 nm, FTIR spectrum was obtained with specific IR ranges of specific functional group. The stretching vibrations at 1110 and 1460 cm^{-1} are attributed to hydroxyl functional groups in polyphenols and phenols. The phenolic group reduce and effectively wrap nanoparticle to prevent them from agglomeration. All of the peaks of stretching vibrations and bends of carboxylic acids, alcoholic groups and polyphenols obtained are similar to the peak discuss by Gomathi et al., 2016 . The size of Ag NPs were observed from SEM analysis it was found to be 180 nm. The wavelength of colloidal suspension with brown color, IR peaks and SEM image obtained confirms the formation of Ag NPs. These values supports the synthesis of stable Ag NPs based on above obtained results.   There was no method reported for determination of Ag NPs from bulk pharmaceuticals by UV spectroscopy. Validated UV spectroscopy was done at 447nm wavelength of Ag NPs. Data of all parameters i.e linearity with R^2 0.995, LOD and LOQ were found to be 18.15 µg/ml and 55 µg/ml respectively, precision with %RSD 0.9% and 0.32%, ruggedness with %RSD 1.32% which were within the limit of <2%. So, from present research work it can be concluded that method is economical, lab scale, accurate, precise, reproducible and validated as per ICH Q2 (R1) guideline. The developed method was found to be having applicability in routine analysis at lab scale even for the validation of in house formulation of the Ag NPs.

ACKNOWLEDGEMENT

The authors wish to acknowledge the Sanjivani College of Pharmaceutical Education and Research, Kopargaon Maharashtra providing generous support and other necessary facilities to carry out this work.

CONFLICT OF INTEREST

No conflict of intreset between any authors

REFERENCES

1. Kamaraj B, Karuppiah M. Green synthesis of Silver Nanoparticles using *Datura metel* leaves extract. Int J Appl Pure Sci Agric 2015;1(3):130–139.

2. Gomathi, M., Rajkumar, P., Prakasam, A. and Ravichandran, K.Green synthesis of Ag NPss using Datura metel leaf extract and assessment of their antibacterial activity. Resource-Efficient Technologies, 2017;3(3) :280–284.

3. Rauwel, P., Küünal, S., Ferdov, S., & Rauwel, E. A review on the green synthesis of Ag NPs and their morphologies studied via SEM. Extreme Mech Lett., 2015.

4. Panáček, A., Kvítek, L., Prucek, R., Kolá, M., Večeová, R., Pizúrová, N. Zboil, R. Silver Colloid Nanoparticles: Synthesis, Characterization, and Their Antibacterial Activity. ChemPhotoChem.2006;110(33):16248–16253.

5. Sharma, K., Agrawal, S. S., & Gupta, M. Development and validation of UV spectrophotometric method for the estimation of curcumin in bulk drug and pharmaceutical dosage forms. Int J Drug Develop 2012;4(2): 375–380.

6. Chaudhari, S., Mannan, A., & Daswadkar, S. Development and validation of UV spectrophotometric method for simultaneous estimation of Acyclovir and Silymarin in niosome formulation. Pharm Lett2016; 8(5):128–133.

7. Patel, J., Kevin, G., Patel, A., Raval, M., & Sheth, N. Development of the UV spectrophotometric method of Olmesartan medoxomil in bulk drug and pharmaceutical formulation and stress degradation studies. Pharm Methods 2016;2(1): 36–41.

8. BOGGULA, . Method development and validations of Apixaban in bulk and its formulations by UV-spectroscopy (area under curve) 2018; 10(3):5617.

9. Chaudhary, H., Kohli, K., Kumar, V., Rathee, S., Rathee, P. A Novel Validated Spectrophotometric Method for Simultaneous Estimation of Diclofenac Diethylamine and Curcumin in Transdermal Gels. Anal Lett2013;1(3): 224–233

10. Behera, S. UV-Visible Spectrophotometric Method Development and Validation of Assay of Paracetamol Tablet Formulation. J Anal Bioanal Tech 2012; 03(06).

11. Umme Bushra, M. U. B. Development and Validation of a Simple UV Spectrophotometric Method for the Determination of Cefotaxime Sodium in Bulk And Pharmaceutical Formulation. IOSR J Pharm (IOSRPHR) 2014; 04(01): 74–77.

12. Chanda, I., Bordoloi, R., Chakraborty, D. D., Chakraborty, P., & Das, S. R. C. Development and validation of UV-spectroscopic method for estimation of niacin in bulk and pharmaceutical dosage form. J Appl Pharm Sci 2017;7(9): 81–84.

13. P. Raveendran, J. Fu, and S. L. Wallen, "Completely "Green" Synthesis and stabilization of metal nanoparticles," *Journal of the American Chemical Society*, 2003;125 (46):13940–13941.

14. J. Kesharwani, K. Y. Yoon, J. Hwang, and M. Rai, "Phytofabrication of silver nanoparticles by leaf extract of Datura metel: hypothetical mechanism involved in synthesis," *Journal of Bionanoscience*,2009: 3,(1): 39–44.

15. J. Kasthuri, K. Kathiravan, and N. Rajendiran, "Phyllanthinassisted biosynthesis of silver and gold nanoparticles: a novel biological approach," *Journal of Nanoparticle Research*, 2009; 11(5):1075–1085.

16. K. Mallikarjuna, G. Narasimha, G. R. Dillip et al. "Green synthesis of silver nanoparticles using *Ocimum leaf* extract and their characterization," *Digest Journal of Nanomaterials and Biostructures*, 2011;8(1):181–186.

17. Ahmed, S., Ahmad, M., Swami, B. L., & Ikram, S.. Plants extract mediated synthesis of silver nanoparticles for antimicrobial applications: a green expertise. Journal of Advance Research.2015

18. Ahmed, S., & Ikram, S.. Chitosan & its derivatives: a review in recent innovations. International Journal of Pharmaceutical Sciences and Research,2015; 6(1): 14–30

19.   Ashokkumar, S., Ravi, S., & Velmurugan, S. Green synthesis of silver nanoparticles from Gloriosa superba L. leaf extract and their catalytic activity. Spectrochimica Acta Part A: Molecular and Biomolecular Spectroscopy, 2013;115:388-392.

20.   Banerjee, P., Satapathy, M., Mukhopahayay, A., & Das, P. Leaf extract mediated green synthesis of silver nanoparticles from widely available Indian plants: synthesis, characterization, antimicrobial property and toxicity analysis. Bioresources and Bioprocessing, 2014; 1(3):1-10.

21.   Bindhu, M. R., & Umadevi,. Antibacterial and catalytic activities of green synthesized silver nanoparticles. Spectrochimica Acta Part A: Molecular and Biomolecular Spectroscopy, 2015;135: 373-378.

22.   Davidson   AG.   Ultraviolet-visible   absorption spectrophotometry. In BeckettAH, Stenlake JB, (4thedn), Practical Pharmaceutical chemistry. CBS Publishers and distributors, New Delhi,2002; 275-278.

TABLE 1: FTIR RANGES OF SYNTHESIZED AG NPS

Observed frequencies (cm⁻¹)	IR Assignments
1046	-C-O- Stretching
1193	-C-O- Stretching
1387	-C-O-C- Stretching
1561	-C-C Stretching
1580	-C-H stretching
1675	-COOH group
1735	-C=O Stretching

TABLE 2 : VALIDATION PARAMETERS OF SYNTHESIZED AG NPS

Parameters	Silver Nanoparticle
Wavelength	447nm
Range	160-660 µg/ml
Linearity equation	Y=0.001x+0.034
R^2	0.995
Slope	0.001
Precision(%R.S.D)	
a) Intraday	0.9%
b) Interday	0.32%
Ruggedness(%R.S.D)	1.23%
LOD	18.15 µg/ml
LOQ	55 µg/ml

TABLE 3: STANDARD GRAPH OF   FLUCONAZOLE

Sr No.	Conc (µg/ml)	Absorbance
1	160	0.242
2	260	0.428
3	360	0.587
4	460	0.726
5	560	0.855
6	660	0.989

TABLE 4: % RECOVERY STUDY OF AG NPS

Level (%)	Amount of AgNPs added(µg/ml)	% recovery	Mean % recovery	% R.S.D
50	160	94.8%	97.7%	0.48%
100	320	99.06%		
150	480	99.24%		

TABLE 5: INTRADAY STUDY OF PRECISION

Sr No.	Conc(μg/ml)	Absorbance	Mean = 0.561 S.D = 0.0055
1	360	0.567	%R.S.D =
2	360	0.556	0.98%
3	360	0.566	
4	360	0.555	
5	360	0.567	
6	360	0.560	

TABLE 6 : INTERDAY STUDY OF PRECISION

Sr No.	Conc(μg/ml)	Absorbance	
			Mean = 0.548
1	360	0.547	
2	360	0.546	S.D =
3	360	0.550	0.0018
4	360	0.546	%R.S.D =
5	360	0.549	0.32%
6	360	0.550	

TABLE 7: RUGGEDNESS STUDY OF AG NPS BY
ANALYST 1

Sr No.	Conc(μg/ml)	Absorbance	Mean = 0.460
			S.D = 0.00568
1	360	0.454	
2	360	0.459	**%R.S.D** =
3	360	0.460	1.23%
4	360	0.458	
5	360	0.460	
6	360	0.471	

TABLE 8: RUGGEDNESS STUDY OF AG NPS
BY ANALYST 2

Sr No.	Conc(μg/ml)	Absorbance	
			Mean =
1	360	0.567	0.561
2	360	0.556	
3	360	0.566	**S.D** =
4	360	0.555	0.0055
5	360	0.567	**%R.S.D**
6	360	0.560	=
			0.98%

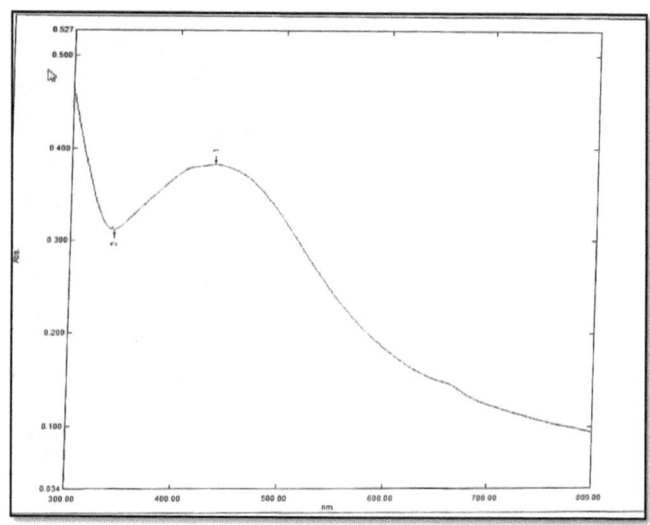

Fig. 1: Ag NPs peak in methanol

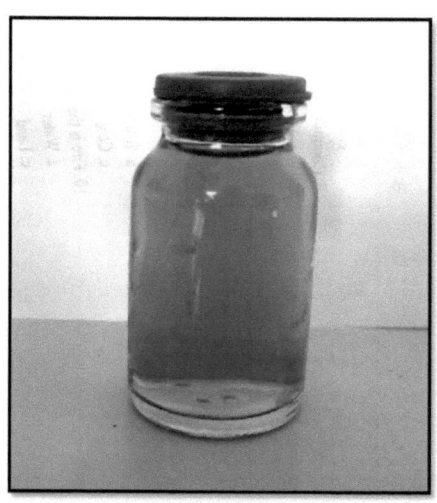

Fig. 2: Colloidal solution of AgNPs

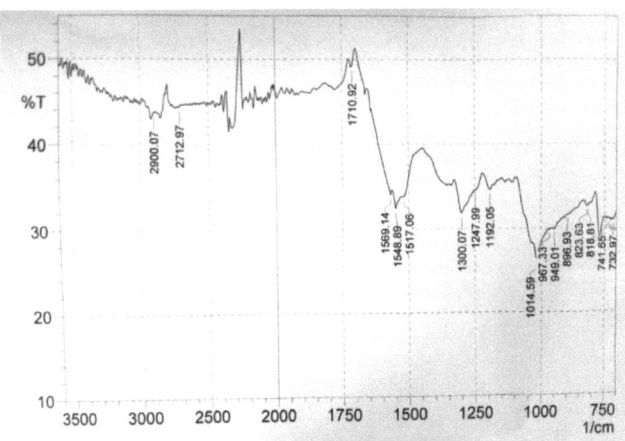

Fig. 3: FTIRspectrum of Ag NPs

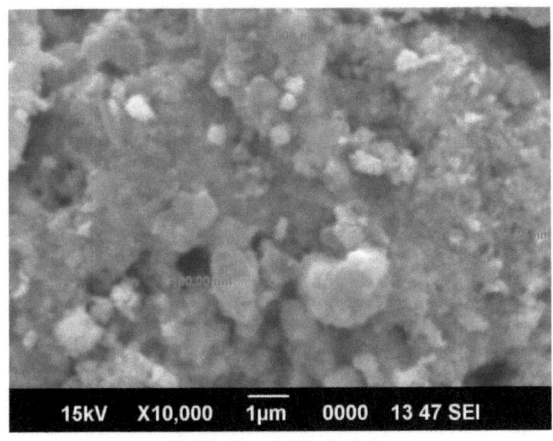

Fig. 4: SEM image of Ag NPs

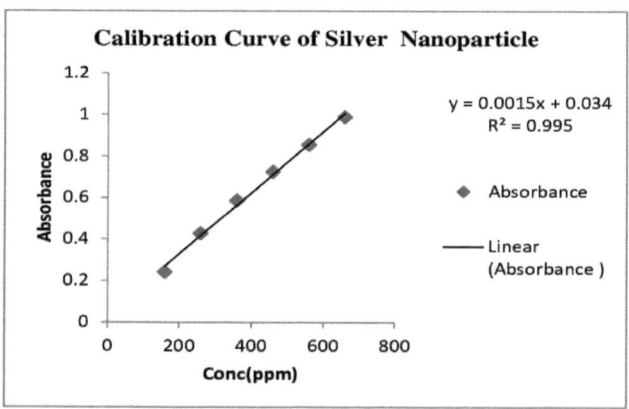

Fig. 5: Calibration curve of Ag NPs in methanol

Table and figure titles and legends:

TABLE 1: FTIR RANGES OF SYNTHESIZED AG NPS

AG NPS stands for silver nanoparticle

TABLE 2: VALIDATION PARAMETERS OF
SYNTHESIZED AG NPS

Include all validation parameters performed for silver
nanoparticle. AG NPS stands for silver nanoparticle

TABLE 3: STANDARD GRAPH OF   FLUCONAZOLE

Concentration in µg/ml along with the absorbance obtained.

TABLE 4 : % RECOVERY STUDY OF AG NPS

SD stand for Standard Deviation, RSD stand for Relative
Standard Deviation .

TABLE 5: INTRADAY STUDY OF PRECISION

Include the study of sample concentration for repetitive time on
the same day. SD stand for Standard Deviation, RSD stand for
Relative Standard Deviation .

TABLE 6: INTERDAY STUDY OF PRECISION

Include the study of sample concentration for repetitive time on
the different day. SD stand for Standard Deviation, RSD stand
for Relative Standard Deviation .

TABLE 7: RUGGEDNESS STUDY OF AG NPS ANALYST 1

SD stand for Standard Deviation, RSD stand for Relative
Standard Deviation. AG NPS stands for silver nanoparticle.
To know the ruggedness of method . Changes on SD
,RSD,%RSD.

TABLE 8: RUGGEDNESS STUDY OF AG NPS ANALYST
2
SD stand for Standard Deviation, RSD stand for Relative
Standard Deviation. AG NPS stands for silver nanoparticle.
To know the ruggedness of method . Changes on SD
,RSD,%RSD by different analyst.

Fig. 1: AgNPs peak in methanol (Author's own work, peak obtain in UV spectroscopy for wavelength)

Ag NPs stand for silver nanoparticle.

Fig.2 : Colloidal solution of Ag NPs (Author's own work, synthesized in laboratory)

Brown color solution indicate silver nanoparticle

Fig.3 : FTIR spectrum of Ag NPs (Author's own work, spectrum obtained from FTIR including presence of various carbonyl group)

FTIR is Fourier Transform Infrared spectrum of silver nanoparticle.

Fig. 4: SEM image of Ag NPs (Author's own work, SEM Analysis to validated the the particles of silver are Nanoparticles or not)

Scanning Electrone Microscopy image of silver nanoparticle in nanometer.

Fig. 5: Calibration curve of As NPs (Author's own work, alidation of AgNPs)

R^2 is regression coefficient of silver nanoparticle in methanol.

YOUR KNOWLEDGE HAS VALUE

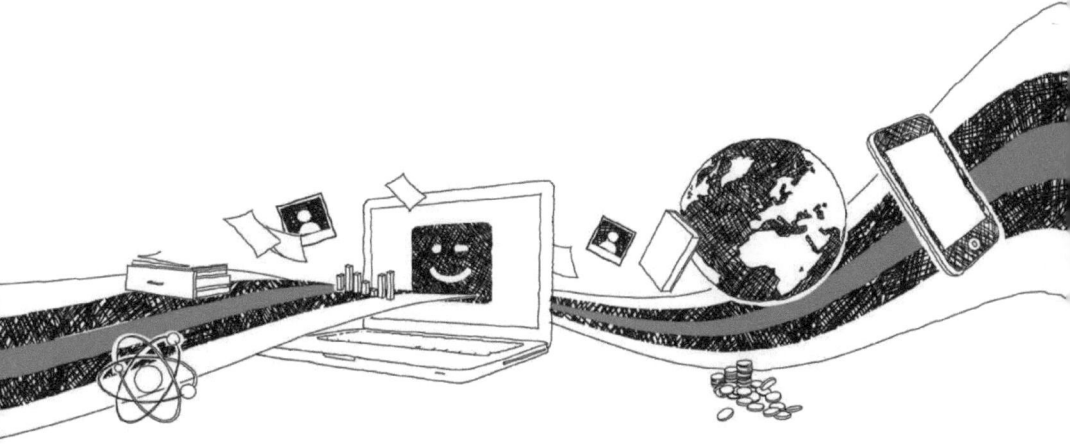

- We will publish your bachelor's and master's thesis, essays and papers

- Your own eBook and book - sold worldwide in all relevant shops

- Earn money with each sale

Upload your text at www.GRIN.com and publish for free

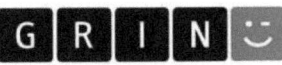